THE KIDNEY

STONE

COOKBOOK

SARAH JACK

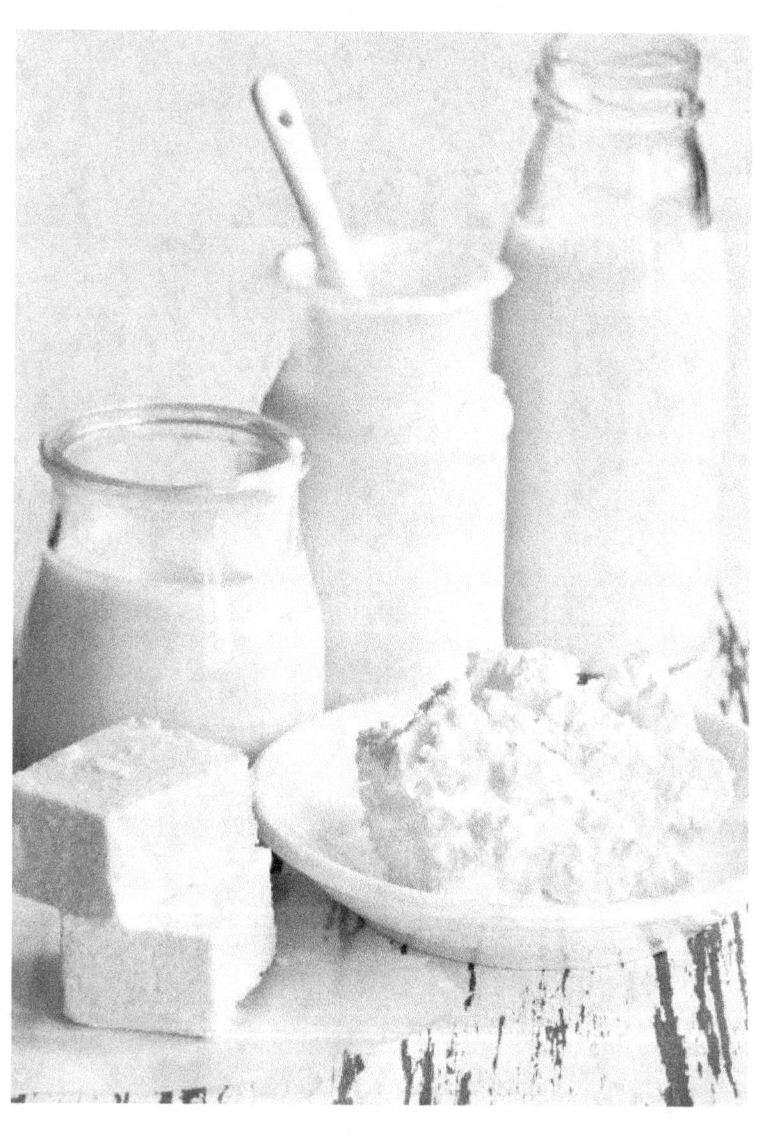

COPYRIGHT

TABLE OF CONTENTS

Table of Contents

COPYRIGHT 3

TABLE OF CONTENTS 4

INTRODUCTION 5

KIDNEY STONE 16

KIDNEY STONE DIET 20

BENEFITS OF KIDNEY STONE DIET 24

KIDNEY STONE DIET RECIPES 28

INTRODUCTION

KIDNEY

The kidneys, two bean-shaped organs nestled in the back of the abdominal cavity, are unsung heroes of the human body. Performing a myriad of vital functions, these organs play a crucial role in maintaining homeostasis and ensuring the body's overall well-being. This exploration delves into the intricate world of kidneys, unraveling their functions, common disorders, preventive measures, and the significance of kidney health in the broader context of human physiology.

- **Anatomy and Location**

The kidneys, paired and symmetrical, are positioned on either side of the spine, just below the ribcage. Protected by layers of muscle and fat, these organs are strategically located to perform their crucial functions efficiently. Each kidney is approximately the size of a fist and is divided into two main regions: the cortex (outer layer) and the medulla (inner region). Renal arteries and veins, responsible for transporting blood to and from the kidneys, are intricately connected to the organ's functioning.

- **Functions of the Kidneys**

Filtration of Blood:

The primary function of the kidneys is to filter the blood, removing waste products and excess substances. This intricate filtration process occurs in tiny units within the kidneys called nephrons. Nephrons filter blood, reabsorbing essential substances (such as water, glucose, and electrolytes) and excreting waste products into urine.

Regulation of Blood Pressure:

The kidneys play a pivotal role in regulating blood pressure. They achieve this by controlling the volume of blood and the concentration of electrolytes. Renin, an enzyme released by the kidneys, stimulates a cascade of reactions that ultimately influence blood pressure.

Acid-Base Balance:

Maintaining the body's acid-base balance is essential for normal cellular function. The kidneys help regulate the acidity of the blood by excreting hydrogen ions and reabsorbing bicarbonate ions.

Erythropoiesis Regulation:

The kidneys produce and release erythropoietin, a hormone that stimulates the production of red blood cells in the bone marrow. This ensures an adequate supply of oxygen to tissues and organs.

Electrolyte Balance:

Sodium, potassium, and other electrolytes are carefully regulated by the kidneys. Imbalances in these electrolytes can have profound effects on nerve function, muscle contraction, and overall cellular activity.

Detoxification:

The kidneys act as a natural detoxifier by filtering and eliminating various toxins, drugs, and metabolic by-products from the bloodstream.

- **Common Kidney Disorders**

Chronic Kidney Disease (CKD):

CKD is a progressive condition where the kidneys gradually lose their function over time. Common causes include hypertension, diabetes, and certain genetic factors. As CKD advances, it can lead to complications such as anemia, bone disease, and cardiovascular issues.

Acute Kidney Injury (AKI):

AKI is a sudden and often reversible loss of kidney function. It can result from conditions like dehydration, severe infections, or exposure to nephrotoxic drugs. Timely intervention is crucial to prevent irreversible damage.

Kidney Stones:

These are hard deposits that form in the kidneys and can cause severe pain when they pass through the urinary tract. Dehydration, diet, and certain medical conditions contribute to the formation of kidney stones.

Urinary Tract Infections (UTIs):

While UTIs can affect any part of the urinary system, including the kidneys, kidney infections (pyelonephritis) specifically target the kidney tissue. Prompt treatment is essential to prevent complications.

Polycystic Kidney Disease (PKD):

PKD is a genetic disorder characterized by the growth of fluid-filled cysts in the kidneys. Over time, these cysts can interfere with normal kidney function, leading to complications.

Glomerulonephritis:

This condition involves inflammation of the glomeruli, the filtering units in the kidneys. It can result from infections, autoimmune diseases, or certain medications.

- **Preventive Measures for Kidney Health**

Hydration:

Adequate water intake is essential for kidney health. It helps flush out toxins and prevents the formation of kidney stones. Maintaining good hydration is especially crucial for those at risk of kidney disorders.

Balanced Diet:

A diet rich in fruits, vegetables, whole grains, and lean proteins contributes to overall health and supports kidney function. Monitoring salt intake is crucial, as excessive salt can contribute to hypertension and kidney damage.

Regular Exercise:

Engaging in regular physical activity promotes cardiovascular health, which is closely linked to kidney function. Exercise also helps control blood pressure and prevent obesity, reducing the risk of kidney disorders.

Blood Sugar Control:

For individuals with diabetes, maintaining optimal blood sugar levels is vital to prevent diabetic nephropathy, a common cause of chronic kidney disease.

Blood Pressure Management:

Hypertension is a leading cause of kidney damage. Regular monitoring of blood pressure and the use of antihypertensive medications when necessary can help preserve kidney function.

Limiting Alcohol and Avoiding Smoking:

Excessive alcohol consumption can impair kidney function, and smoking has been linked to an increased risk of kidney cancer. Avoiding or moderating these habits contributes to overall kidney health.

- **Diagnostic Techniques and Treatment Options**

Blood Tests:

Blood tests, such as serum creatinine and blood urea nitrogen (BUN), provide indicators of kidney function. Elevated levels may suggest kidney impairment.

Urinalysis:

Examining the urine can reveal signs of kidney disorders, such as the presence of blood, protein, or abnormal cells.

Imaging Studies:

Ultrasound, CT scans, and MRIs are used to visualize the structure of the kidneys and identify abnormalities, such as cysts, stones, or tumors.

Biopsy:

In some cases, a kidney biopsy may be performed to assess tissue damage and guide treatment decisions.

Medications:

Depending on the underlying cause of kidney disorders, medications may be prescribed to manage blood pressure, reduce inflammation, or treat infections.

Dialysis and Kidney Transplant:

In cases of advanced kidney failure, dialysis or kidney transplantation may be necessary. Dialysis involves using a machine to filter and cleanse the blood when the kidneys can no longer perform this function adequately.

- **Conclusion:**

The kidneys, often overlooked in their quiet efficiency, are integral to the body's equilibrium. From filtration and regulation to detoxification and erythropoiesis, their functions are diverse and indispensable. Understanding the complexities of kidney health, being aware of preventive measures, and recognizing the signs of potential disorders are paramount for maintaining overall well-being.

In the intricate interplay of bodily functions, the kidneys stand as vigilant custodians, contributing to the symphony of life. As we navigate the complexities of modern living, cultivating an awareness of kidney health becomes not only a necessity but a celebration of the remarkable resilience and intricacy of the human body. It is a call to action, urging us to care for these unsung heroes and appreciate the profound impact they have on our vitality, longevity, and the delicate balance of our existence.

KIDNEY STONE

Kidney stones are solid deposits of minerals and salts that develop inside the kidneys and are referred to medically as nephrolithiasis or renal calculi. They can range in size from being the size of a golf ball to a grain of sand. Kidney stones can be excruciatingly painful and may result in a variety of symptoms, such as:

- An acute, cramp-like discomfort in the side or lower back, frequently extending to the lower abdomen and groin, is the most typical sign of kidney stones. This ache is frequently cited as among the worst ones a person can go through.

- Hematuria: Another typical indication of kidney stones is blood in the urine. Blood in the urine can cause it to appear pink, red, or brown.

- Urination on a regular basis: People with kidney stones may experience an increased need to urinate on a regular basis.

- Urination that hurts: Passing a kidney stone can hurt, possibly resulting in a burning feeling or discomfort.

- Urine that is cloudy or smells bad: Kidney stones can occasionally alter the color or smell of urine.

- Vomiting and nauseousness: Kidney stone pain occasionally causes nauseousness and vomiting.

When specific elements in the urine, such as calcium, oxalate, and uric acid, concentrate and crystallize, kidney stones can develop. A solid mass can then be created by combining these crystals. Depending on the precise minerals involved, there are many forms of kidney stones.

The type of treatment for kidney stones depends on the size, location, and intensity of the symptoms of the condition. Typical forms of treatment include:

- Pain management: Nonsteroidal anti-inflammatory medications (NSAIDs) or opioids may be recommended as treatments for pain.

- Fluid intake: It's important to stay hydrated to wash away kidney stones of a smaller size. Drinking more water can also aid in reducing the likelihood of developing stones later on.

- Drugs: Depending on the type of kidney stone, drugs may be recommended to aid in the dissolution or stop the development of stones.

- Extracorporeal Shock Wave Lithotripsy (ESWL): This method employs shock waves to fragment kidney stones, allowing them to flow through the body more easily.

- In order to remove or dislodge stones from the ureter or kidney, a tiny tube containing a camera is inserted via the urethra and bladder.

- Surgery: The removal of the stones may be required in situations where other treatments are ineffective or the stones are particularly large.

Maintaining a healthy level of hydration, making dietary modifications (limited high-oxalate foods, moderating calcium consumption, and reducing sodium), and controlling underlying medical disorders that raise the risk of stone formation are all effective kidney stone prevention measures. It's critical to get medical help as soon as possible for a suitable diagnosis and course of treatment if you feel you may have kidney stones or suffer severe symptoms.

KIDNEY STONE DIET

A kidney stone diet focuses on dietary modifications that can help prevent kidney stone formation or lower the risk of recurrent kidney stones. Depending on the sort of kidney stones you are prone to developing (such as calcium oxalate stones, uric acid stones, etc.), the specific advice may change. For individualized advice, it's essential to speak with a medical expert or a registered dietitian who can evaluate your unique circumstances and make customized dietary suggestions. However, the following general dietary recommendations are frequently given for avoiding kidney stones:

- Keep Hydrated: Proper hydration is one of the most important elements of kidney stone prevention. By hydrating properly, minerals and salts are less prone to accumulate and form stones in the urine. If you live in a hot area or are prone to kidney stones, aim for at least 8 to 10 cups (64 to 80 ounces) of water per day.

- Limit Your Sodium (Salt) Intake: High sodium intake raises your chance of developing kidney stones that contain calcium. Limit your intake of packaged and processed foods, which are frequently rich in salt. Try to limit your daily sodium intake to 2,300 milligrams or less.

- Moderate Calcium consumption: Although it may seem paradoxical, it's important to maintain a sufficient but moderate calcium consumption. Over supplements, calcium from food sources is favored. Dairy products are a great source of dietary calcium, including yogurt and low-fat milk.

- Watch meals High in Oxalates: If you have calcium oxalate stones, you may need to limit oxalate-rich meals because they can cause stone development. Spinach, rhubarb, beets, sweet potatoes, almonds, and tea are some foods high in oxalate. It could be important to decrease your consumption of certain items.

- Limit your intake of animal proteins: Red meat in particular can raise your chance of developing some kidney stones. Think about including more tofu, beans, and other plant-based protein sources in your diet.

- Moderate Purine-Rich meals: It's vital to cut back on meals high in purines if you have uric acid stones, which are associated with high amounts of uric acid in the urine. These include shellfish, some fish, and organ meats. Keeping alcohol and sugary drinks to a minimum can also aid in lowering uric acid levels.

- Increase Citrus Fruits: Citrus fruits contain a lot of citrate, which can help stop the production of stones. Examples of citrus fruits include lemons, oranges, and limes. Think about increasing your intake of citrus fruits or using lemon juice in your drink.

- Control Portion proportions: Watch your portion proportions because eating too much of some foods, including those that are thought to be healthy, can raise your risk of developing stones. Include a variety of items from various food categories in your diet to maintain balance.

- Monitor Your Urine: If you have a history of kidney stones, your doctor may advise routine urine testing to look for conditions that could lead to the production of stones. This may influence your eating decisions.

Keep in mind that depending on the sort of kidney stones you've had and your general health, different dietary advice may apply to you. Working with a healthcare expert or qualified dietitian to develop a custom kidney stone prevention strategy that meets your unique requirements and preferences is crucial.

BENEFITS OF KIDNEY STONE DIET

A kidney stone diet, which is intended to stop the development of kidney stones or lower the risk of repeated stones, may have the following advantages:

- Reduces the Risk of Kidney Stones: The main advantage of a kidney stone diet is a decreased risk of kidney stone development. You can lessen the risk of stone development by changing your diet to help control the amount of minerals and salts in your urine.

- Reduces discomfort and Discomfort: When kidney stones move through the urinary tract, they can cause terrible discomfort. The development of larger stones, which are more likely to cause excruciating pain and agony during passage, can be avoided by adhering to a kidney stone diet.

- Avoids the Need for Surgery: Kidney stones occasionally need to be removed through surgery. You may be able to avoid the need for surgery and all of the risks and expenses that go along with it by controlling your diet and using preventative measures.

- Improves Hydration: A kidney stone diet's main element is enough hydration. In addition to preventing the formation of stones, adequate hydration promotes general health and wellbeing. Maintaining enough hydration is important for kidney health and can aid in the removal of waste products and toxins from the body.

- Encourages Healthy Eating Habits: A kidney stone diet frequently calls for choosing healthier foods. This may entail consuming fewer processed foods, sugary drinks, and large amounts of sodium while consuming more fruits, vegetables, and other nutrient-dense foods. The management of weight and lowered risk of chronic diseases are just two additional health advantages that may result from these dietary adjustments.

- Customized Approach: Depending on the sort of kidney stones you've had and your unique risk factors, a kidney stone diet can be made to suit your individual needs. Your diet will be specifically tailored to fit your individual needs if you work with a healthcare provider or certified dietician.

- Increased Awareness: Adopting a kidney stone diet frequently calls for people to increase their awareness of their food choices and the effects of particular foods on their health. Better long-term eating habits and an increase in general health consciousness may result from this increased knowledge.

- May Enhance Bone Health: It's critical to maintain an optimal level of calcium in your diet to support bone health, despite worries about calcium intake and kidney stones. You may help guarantee that you receive the proper amount of calcium without raising your risk of stone development by following a kidney stone diet that is well-balanced.

It's important to understand that a kidney stone diet's efficiency varies depending on the type of stones you've had and your unique risk factors. Always follow dietary guidelines with the help of a medical expert or certified dietitian who can offer tailored counseling and keep track of your progress. To significantly lower the chance of kidney stones, it's also critical to combine dietary modifications with other preventive measures, such as drinking enough of water and taking any prescribed medications.

KIDNEY STONE DIET RECIPES

Lemon-Herb Grilled Chicken

Ingredients

- 4 skinless, boneless breasts of chicken

- 2 lemons (juiced and zested)

- 2 minced garlic cloves

- 2 teaspoons chopped fresh rosemary

- 2 teaspoons chopped fresh thyme

- Pepper and salt as desired

Instructions:

- Lemon juice, lemon zest, minced garlic, rosemary, thyme, salt, and pepper should be combined in a bowl to make a marinade.

- Place chicken breasts in a resealable bag or dish and pour the marinade over them. Seal and refrigerate for at least 30 minutes.

- Preheat a grill to medium-high heat.

- Grill chicken for 6 to 8 minutes on each side, or until done.

Creamy Cauliflower Soup

Ingredients:

- 1 head cauliflower (cut into florets)

- One small onion, diced

- 2 minced garlic cloves

- 4 cups of vegetable broth low in salt

- 1 cup plain Greek yogurt with low fat

- Pepper and salt as desired

- Chopped fresh parsley (for garnish)

Instructions:

- Sliced onion and minced garlic should be softened in a big pot with a little olive oil.

- Vegetable broth and cauliflower florets should be added to the pot. Bring to a boil before turning down the heat and simmering the cauliflower for a while.

- To purée the soup, use an immersion blender or a standard blender.

- Add Greek yogurt to the soup before adding it back to the pot. Do not boil, just gently heat.

- To taste, add salt and pepper to the food.

- Serve hot with freshly chopped parsley as a garnish.

Strawberry and Spinach Salad

Ingredients:

- 4 cups fresh leaves of spinach

- 1 cup of strawberry slices

- A quarter cup of toasted almond slices

- 2 tablespoons balsamic vinaigrette dressing (low in sodium)

Instructions:

- Sliced strawberries, fresh spinach, and toasted sliced almonds should all be combined in a big bowl.

- Drizzle with balsamic vinaigrette dressing.

- Gently toss the salad to evenly distribute the dressing over the items.

- Serve the salad as a refreshing side dish.

Roasted Vegetable Medley

Ingredients:

- 2 cups mixed vegetables (such as zucchini, bell peppers, and cherry tomatoes)

- 2 tablespoons olive oil

- 2 cloves garlic (minced)

- 1 teaspoon dried oregano

- Pepper and salt as desired

Instructions:

- Set the oven's temperature to 425°F (220°C).

- Mixtures of veggies should be blended with olive oil, minced garlic, dried oregano, salt, and pepper in a big bowl.

- On a baking sheet, arrange the vegetables in a single layer.

- The veggies should be roasted in the preheated oven for 20 to 25 minutes, or until they are soft and just beginning to caramelize.

Watermelon and Cucumber Salad

Ingredients:

- 4 cups of watermelon cubes

- 1 cucumber, sliced

- Feta cheese crumbles, 1/4 cup (optional)

- Leaves of fresh mint (for garnish)

- Balsamic glaze (low in sodium, for drizzling)

Instructions:

- Cubed watermelon and thinly sliced cucumber should be combined in a big bowl.

- Add some feta cheese crumbles if you like.

- Use fresh mint leaves as a garnish.

- To add flavor, drizzle with balsamic glaze.

Grilled Portobello Mushrooms

Ingredients:

- Large Portobello mushrooms, four,

- 2 tablespoons low-sodium balsamic vinegar

- Olive oil, two tablespoons

- 2 minced garlic cloves

- Pepper and salt as desired

- Fresh basil leaves (for garnish)

Instructions:

- Set the grill's temperature to medium-high.

- Balsamic vinegar, olive oil, minced garlic, salt, and pepper should all be combined in a small bowl.

- The balsamic mixture should be applied to the Portobello mushrooms' both surfaces.

- The mushrooms should be grilled until soft, about 4-5 minutes per side.

- Before serving, garnish with fresh basil leaves.

Brown Rice and Black Bean Salad

Ingredients:

- 2 cups of cooked and cooled brown rice

- 1 can (15 ounces) of rinsed and drained black beans

- 1 cup thawed corn kernels, either fresh or frozen

- 1 chopped red bell pepper

- 1/4 cup finely chopped red onion

- 1/2 cup chopped fresh cilantro

- Lime juice, 2 tablespoons

- Olive oil, two tablespoons

- 1 teaspoon of cumin, ground

- Pepper and salt as desired

- Avocado slices (optional garnish)

Instructions:

- Cooked brown rice, black beans, corn kernels, red bell pepper, red onion, finely diced, and fresh cilantro should all be combined in a big bowl.

- In a separate small bowl, whisk together lime juice, olive oil, ground cumin, salt, and pepper to make the dressing.

- After adding the dressing, toss the salad to incorporate.

- Garnish with avocado slices if desired.

Turkey and Vegetable Skewers

Ingredients:

- 1-pound lean turkey breast (cut into cubes)

- 2 bell peppers (cut into chunks)

- 1 red onion (cut into chunks)

- Olive oil, two tablespoons

- Lemon juice, two tablespoons

- 1 teaspoon dried oregano

- Pepper and salt as desired

Instructions:

- Cubed turkey breast, bell pepper chunks, red onion chunks, olive oil, lemon juice, dried oregano, salt, and pepper should all be combined in a bowl. Coat by tossing.

- Thread the turkey and vegetable pieces onto skewers.

- Preheat a grill to medium-high heat.

- The skewers should be grilled on the grill for 10 to 12 minutes, turning them once, or until the turkey is thoroughly cooked.

Baked Cod with Herbs

Ingredients:

- 4 cod fillets

- Olive oil, two tablespoons

- 2 minced garlic cloves

- 2 teaspoons freshly chopped parsley

- 1 tablespoon chopped fresh dill

- Pepper and salt as desired

- Lemon wedges (for serving)

Instructions:

- Set the oven's temperature to 375°F (190°C).

- Cod fillets should be placed on a baking pan covered lined parchment paper. Olive oil should be drizzled over the dish before being seasoned with salt, pepper, minced garlic, fresh parsley, and fresh dill.

- Bake for 15 to 20 minutes in a preheated oven, or until the cod flakes easily with a fork.

- Lemon wedges should be served on the side.

Blueberry Oatmeal Pancakes

Ingredients:

- Old-fashioned oats, 1 cup

- Low-fat Greek yogurt, half a cup

- Two ripe bananas

- 2 eggs

- One-half teaspoon of vanilla extract

- One tablespoon of baking powder

- 1/2 cups of fresh or frozen blueberries

- Cooking spray (for the pan)

Instructions:

- Put eggs, vanilla extract, baking powder, old-fashioned oats, low-fat Greek yogurt, ripe bananas, and into a blender. Blend the batter up to smoothness.

- Fold the blueberries gently into the batter.

- Heat a non-stick skillet over medium heat and lightly grease it with cooking spray.

- Pour pancake batter onto the skillet to form pancakes of your desired size.

- Cook until surface bubbles appear, then turn and continue to cook the other side until golden.

- Serve with more blueberries and a dollop of low-fat Greek yogurt.

Zucchini Noodles with Pesto

Ingredients:

- 4 medium zucchinis (spiralized into noodles)

- 1 cup of basil leaves, fresh

- 1/4 cup roasted pine nuts

- Garlic cloves, two

- Grated Parmesan cheese, 1/4 cup

- Olive oil, 1/4 cup

- Pepper and salt as desired

- Cherry tomatoes (optional garnish)

Instructions:

- Fresh basil, toasted pine nuts, minced garlic, grated Parmesan cheese, extra virgin olive oil, salt, and pepper are all combined in a food processor. Blend until a smooth pesto sauce is achieved.

- A little olive oil should be heated up in a big skillet over medium heat. Add the zucchini noodles and cook for an additional two to three minutes, or until just tender.

- Combine the pesto sauce with the zucchini noodles.

- If desired, add cherry tomatoes as a garnish before serving.

Grilled Shrimp and Vegetable Skewers

Ingredients:

- 1-pound large shrimp (peeled and deveined)

- 2 bell peppers (cut into chunks)

- 1 sliced zucchini

- 1 red onion (cut into chunks)

- 2 minced garlic cloves

- Olive oil, two tablespoons

- One teaspoon of lemon juice

- 1 teaspoon dried oregano

- Pepper and salt as desired

Instructions:

- Shrimp that has been peeled and deveined, bell pepper pieces, zucchini slices, red onion chunks, minced garlic, olive oil, lemon juice, dried oregano, salt, and pepper should all be combined in a bowl. Coat by tossing.

- The shrimp and veggie pieces are skewered together.

- Grill at a medium-high temperature.

- About 3 to 4 minutes should be spent grilling each side of the skewers until the shrimp are done and pink.

Turkey and Vegetable Stir-Fry with Brown Rice

Ingredients:

- 1 pound of turkey, ground

- 2 cups mixed vegetables (such as broccoli, bell peppers, and snap peas)

- 2 minced garlic cloves

- Low-sodium soy sauce, two tablespoons

- One teaspoon of sesame oil

- 1 teaspoon of minced ginger

- Cooked brown rice (for serving)

Instructions:

- Cook ground turkey in a pan over a medium heat until browned. Drain any excess fat.

- Add minced garlic and a mixture of veggies to the skillet. Stir-fry until vegetables are tender but still crisp.

- Low-sodium soy sauce, sesame oil, and minced ginger are combined in a small bowl.

- Pour the sauce over the turkey and vegetable mixture and stir to combine.

- Serve over cooked brown rice.

Cauliflower Rice Pilaf

Ingredients:

- 1 head cauliflower (cut into florets)

- 1/2 cup chopped onion

- 1/2 cup chopped bell pepper (red or green)

- A half-cup of chopped celery

- 1 cup of carrots, chopped

- 2 minced garlic cloves

- Olive oil, two tablespoons

- a half-teaspoon of dried thyme

- A half-teaspoon of dried rosemary

- Pepper and salt as desired

- Chopped fresh parsley (for garnish)

Instructions:

- In a food processor, pulse cauliflower florets until they resemble rice grains. Place aside.

- Olive oil should be heated in a big skillet over a medium heat. Add chopped celery, carrot, onion, bell pepper, and garlic. Sauté until vegetables are tender.

- Add the cauliflower rice, salt, pepper, dried thyme, and dried rosemary. Cook for a further 5-7 minutes, stirring occasionally.

- Garnish with chopped fresh parsley before serving.

Lemon-Garlic Grilled Chicken

Ingredients:

- 4 skinless, boneless breasts of chicken

- 2 lemons (juiced)

- 4 minced garlic cloves

- 2 teaspoons freshly chopped parsley

- Olive oil, two tablespoons

- Pepper and salt as desired

Instructions:

- To make a marinade, combine the lemon juice, garlic powder, fresh parsley, olive oil, salt, and pepper in a basin.

- Put the marinade over the chicken breasts in a dish or resealable bag. Seal and refrigerate for at least 30 minutes.

- Preheat a grill to medium-high heat.

- Grill chicken for 6 to 8 minutes on each side, or until done.

Spaghetti Squash with Tomato Sauce

Ingredients:

- Spaghetti squash, one

- 2 cups of tomato sauce low in salt

- Olive oil, 1 tbsp

- 2 minced garlic cloves

- One tablespoon dried basil

- 1 teaspoon dried oregano

- Pepper and salt as desired

- Fresh basil leaves (for garnish)

Instructions:

- Set the oven's temperature to 375°F (190°C).

- Scoop out the seeds after cutting the spaghetti squash in half lengthwise.

- Place the squash halves, cut side down, on a baking sheet and roast in the preheated oven for about 40-45 minutes or until the flesh is tender.

- While the squash is roasting, heat olive oil in a saucepan over medium heat. Add minced garlic and sauté until fragrant.

- Stir in low-sodium tomato sauce, dried basil, dried oregano, salt, and pepper. Simmer for a few minutes.

- When the spaghetti squash is finished cooking, use a fork to scrape the flesh into "noodles."

- Serve the squash noodles with the tomato sauce and garnish with fresh basil leaves.

Roasted Beet and Goat Cheese Salad

Ingredients:

- 4 medium beets, peeled and diced

- Olive oil, two tablespoons

- Pepper and salt as desired

- 4 cups mixed greens (such as arugula and spinach)

- 1/2 cup crumbled goat cheese

- A quarter cup of roasted walnuts

- Balsamic glaze (low in sodium, for drizzling)

Instructions:

- Set the oven's temperature to 400°F (200°C).

- Toss diced beets with olive oil, salt, and pepper, and spread them in a single layer on a baking sheet.

- Roast in the preheated oven for about 30-35 minutes or until the beets are tender.

- Place mixed greens in a big bowl and garnish with roasted beets, goat cheese that has been crumbled, and toasted walnuts.

- Before serving, drizzle with balsamic glaze.

White Bean and Tuna Salad

Ingredients:

- 2 cans (5 ounces each) tuna in water (drained)

- 1 can (15 ounces) white beans (cannellini or Great Northern, drained and rinsed)

- 1/4 cup finely chopped red onion

- 1/4 cup chopped fresh parsley

- Lemon juice, two tablespoons

- Olive oil, two tablespoons

- Pepper and salt as desired

Instructions:

- Drained tuna, white beans, finely chopped red onion, fresh parsley, lemon juice, olive oil, salt, and pepper should all be combined in a big bowl.

- Combine by tossing.

- Serve chilled as a hearty salad.

Baked Eggplant Parmesan

Ingredients:

- 2 large eggplants (sliced into rounds)

- 2 cups low-sodium marinara sauce

- 1 cup of shredded part-skim mozzarella cheese

- Grated Parmesan cheese, 1/4 cup

- Olive oil, two tablespoons

- Whole wheat breadcrumbs in a cup

- A quarter cup of chopped fresh basil leaves

- Pepper and salt as desired

Instructions:

- Set the oven's temperature to 375°F (190°C).

- Place eggplant slices on a baking sheet and brush both sides with olive oil. Season with salt and pepper.

- Combine breadcrumbs, Parmesan cheese, and fresh basil in a small dish.

- Dredge each eggplant slice in the breadcrumb mixture, pressing lightly to adhere.

- The coated eggplant slices should be baked for 20 to 25 minutes, or until they are soft and golden brown, on a baking sheet in a preheated oven.

- Place half of the roasted eggplant slices, half of the marinara sauce, and half of the mozzarella cheese in a baking dish. Repeat the layers.

- Bake the cheese for a further 15 to 20 minutes, or until bubbling and brown.

- Serve Hot.

Lemon-Garlic Shrimp Scampi

Ingredients:

- 1 pound large shrimp (peeled and deveined)

- 8 ounces of whole-wheat pasta

- Olive oil, two tablespoons

- 4 minced garlic cloves

- Two lemons' juice and zest

- 1/4 cup chopped fresh parsley

- Pepper and salt as desired

Instructions:

- Follow the directions on the package to prepare the whole wheat linguine. Drain, then set apart.

- Olive oil should be heated in a big skillet over a medium heat. Sauté garlic till aromatic after adding.

- Peeled and deveined shrimp should be added to the skillet and cooked for two to three minutes on each side, or until pink and opaque.

- Toss the cooked linguine with the shrimp mixture and serve hot.

Mixed Berry Chia Seed Pudding

Ingredients:

- 1 cup mixed berries (such as strawberries, blueberries, and raspberries)

- 1/4 cup chia seeds

- 1 cup unsweetened almond milk

- 1 tablespoon honey (optional)

Instructions:

- Blend the mixed berries, chia seeds, almond milk without added sugar, and honey, if using, in a blender. Until smooth, blend.

- Fill separate jars or a basin with the mixture.

- Refrigerate the pudding for at least two to three hours, or until it has thickened.

- If desired, top with more berries when serving cold.

Chicken Skewers with Cilantro and Lime

Ingredients:

- 1-pound boneless, skinless chicken breasts (cut into cubes)

- 2 cloves garlic (minced)

- Zest and juice of 2 limes

- 1/4 cup fresh cilantro (chopped)

- Olive oil, two tablespoons

- pepper and salt as desired

Instructions:

- To make a marinade, mix the minced garlic, olive oil, lime zest, lime juice, chopped cilantro, salt, and pepper in a basin.

- Place chicken cubes in a resealable bag or dish and pour the marinade over them. Seal and refrigerate for at least 30 minutes.

- Grill at a medium-high temperature.

- Chicken chunks that have been marinated are skewered.

- Cook the chicken on the skewers on the grill for about 4-5 minutes on each side, or until done.

Cauliflower and Broccoli Bake

Ingredients:

- 1 head of floretized cauliflower

- 1 head of floretized broccoli

- Olive oil, two tablespoons

- 2 minced garlic cloves

- Grated Parmesan cheese, 1/4 cup

- pepper and salt as desired

- Freshly chopped parsley

Instructions:

- Set the oven's temperature to 375°F (190°C).

- Cauliflower and broccoli florets, olive oil, minced garlic, salt, and pepper are all combined in a big bowl. Coat by tossing.

- On a baking sheet, arrange the broccoli and cauliflower in a single layer.

- The veggies should be cooked in the preheated oven for 20 to 25 minutes, or until they are soft.

- Before serving, top with freshly chopped parsley and grated Parmesan cheese.

Spinach and Mushroom Quiche

Ingredients:

- 1 whole wheat pie crust, prepared

- 1 prepared whole wheat pie crust

- 1 cup fresh spinach leaves

- 1 cup mushrooms (sliced)

- 1/2 cup diced onion

- 4 eggs

- 1 cup low-fat milk

- 1/2 cup shredded low-fat cheese (such as Swiss or mozzarella)

Instructions:

- Set the oven's temperature to 375°F (190°C).

- Sliced mushrooms and diced onion should be cooked until soft in a skillet. Add some more spinach leaves and cook them until they wilt. Add salt and pepper to taste.

- Whisk eggs and low-fat milk together in a bowl.

- In the whole wheat pie crust that has been prepared, add the sautéed vegetables. Pour the egg and milk mixture over the vegetables and cheese.

- Over the cheese and vegetables, pour the egg and milk mixture.

- For about 30-35 minutes, or until the quiche is set and slightly browned, bake in the preheated oven.

Sweet Potato and Black Bean Chili

Ingredients:

- 2 sweet potatoes (peeled and diced)

- 1 can (15 ounces) black beans (drained and rinsed)

- 1 can (15 ounces) diced tomatoes (low in sodium)

- 1 cup vegetable broth (low-sodium)

- 1 onion (chopped)

- 2 cloves garlic (minced)

- 1 tablespoon chili powder

- 1 teaspoon cumin

- 1 teaspoon paprika

- Salt and pepper to taste

- Olive oil for cooking

- Fresh cilantro is optionally used as a garnish.

Instructions:

- Sliced onion and minced garlic should be softened in a big pot with a little olive oil.

- Spice up the dish by adding diced sweet potatoes, drained black beans, diced tomatoes, vegetable broth, chili powder, cumin, and paprika. When the sweet potatoes are ready, simmer after bringing to a boil.

- Serve hot, garnished with fresh cilantro if desired.

Quinoa Salad with Cucumber and Mint

Ingredients:

- 1 cup quinoa, cooked

- 1 cucumber, diced

- 1/4 cup fresh mint, chopped

- 2 tablespoons olive oil

- Juice of 1 lemon

- Salt and pepper to taste

Instructions:

- In a bowl, combine quinoa, cucumber, and mint.

- Whisk together olive oil, lemon juice, salt, and pepper.

- Pour dressing over the quinoa mixture and toss.

Baked Salmon with Dill

Ingredients:

- 4 salmon fillets

- 2 tablespoons fresh dill, chopped

- 1 tablespoon olive oil

- 1 lemon, sliced

- Salt and pepper to taste

Instructions:

- Preheat oven to 375°F (190°C).

- Place salmon fillets on a baking sheet.

- Drizzle with olive oil, sprinkle with dill, and season with salt and pepper.

- Top with lemon slices and bake for 15-20 minutes or until cooked through.

Cauliflower and Broccoli Stir-Fry

Ingredients:

- 2 cups cauliflower florets

- 2 cups broccoli florets

- 1 tablespoon sesame oil

- 2 tablespoons low-sodium soy sauce

- 1 teaspoon ginger, minced

- 1 teaspoon garlic, minced

Instructions:

- Heat sesame oil in a wok or pan.

- Add cauliflower and broccoli and stir-fry until tender.

- Mix in soy sauce, ginger, and garlic. Stir well and serve.

Watermelon and Feta Salad

Ingredients:

- 4 cups watermelon, cubed

- 1 cup feta cheese, crumbled

- 1/4 cup fresh mint, chopped

- Balsamic glaze for drizzling

Instructions:

- In a large bowl, combine watermelon, feta, and mint.

- Drizzle with balsamic glaze before serving.

Brown Rice Pilaf with Asparagus

Ingredients:

- 1 cup brown rice, cooked

- 1 bunch asparagus, trimmed and chopped

- 1 tablespoon olive oil

- 2 cloves garlic, minced

- 1/4 cup pine nuts

- Salt and pepper to taste

Instructions:

- In a pan, sauté garlic in olive oil.

- Add asparagus and cook until tender.

- Stir in cooked brown rice, pine nuts, salt, and pepper.

Greek Yogurt Parfait

Ingredients:

- 1 cup Greek yogurt

- 1/2 cup granola

- 1/2 cup mixed berries

- 1 tablespoon honey

Instructions:

- In a glass, layer Greek yogurt, granola, and berries.

- Drizzle with honey before serving.

Avocado and Tomato Salsa

Ingredients:

- 2 avocados, diced

- 1 cup cherry tomatoes, halved

- 1/4 cup red onion, finely chopped

- 1 jalapeño, seeded and minced

- 2 tablespoons fresh cilantro, chopped

- Juice of 1 lime

- Salt and pepper to taste

Instructions:

- In a bowl, combine avocados, tomatoes, red onion, jalapeño, and cilantro.

- Drizzle with lime juice and season with salt and pepper.

Baked Sweet Potato Fries

Ingredients:

- 2 sweet potatoes, cut into fries

- 2 tablespoons olive oil

- 1 teaspoon paprika

- 1/2 teaspoon garlic powder

- Salt and pepper to taste

Instructions:

- Preheat oven to 425°F (220°C).

- Toss sweet potato fries with olive oil, paprika, garlic powder, salt, and pepper.

- Bake until golden and crispy.

THANKS FOR READING THIS BOOK.